THE 14-DAY SHIFT
Naturopathic Body Health

THE DIVINE PROTOCOL
FIT FOR THE KINGDOM

YOLANDA O. GREER

The Divine Protocol: Fit for The Kingdom (The 14-Day Shift)
Naturopathic Body Health

Entire contents by Yolanda O. Greer, Founder & Author

San Antonio, Texas

Printed in U.S.A.

Table of Contents

LOVING YOUR BODY

Our goal is to empower the Body of Christ in deliverance for their physical bodies, to bring the triune man into alignment with the Kingdom of God through Naturopathic Body Health. Understanding that the body is equally as powerful as the spirit and the soul, they each work as one with different functionalities. The body should no longer be overlooked during the deliverance process as we renew and cleanse our soul with the Word of God, the body must undergo a cleansing process simultaneously to bring it to its optimal state of dominion.

What I have noticed in the area of deliverance with the Body of Christ, most are focused on the spirit and the soul, with no emphasis on the body. This may potentially leave the body accessible to our enemy (Satan). He hates that we even have bodies because they are a reminder of God's image (*Genesis 1:27*), so he seeks to destroy it with disease, high blood pressure, diabetes, heart problems, etc. The human body is a portal. According to Merriam-Webster, a portal is defined as 1 a door, entrance especially: a grand or imposing one. The body is the one thing that we have that will always rebel against submission, authority, and alignment (*Romans 8:7, 7:23*). Therefore, we are responsible for the whole triune man, when the mind is renewed the body must follow. And this is done when we take dominion over our physical bodies through deliverance by way of healthy eating— changing the way we think about what we consume daily.

"And not only they, but ourselves also, which have the first fruits of the Spirit, even we ourselves grown within ourselves, waiting for the adoption, to wit, the redemption of our body."
—Romans 8:23 KJV

We should be as sensitive to our bodies as we are to our spirit and soul, resisting anything that could cause us harm and keep us physically bound. We are made whole as we shift our perspective— no longer distracted by the enemy with self-esteem issues, sickness, diseases, or any other thing that he seeks to provoke or produce in thought. I am passionate about my desire to give the Body of Christ a jump start into understanding truly what the body needs and uses to begin to bring about complete deliverance. I created The Divine Protocol to help bring support to our physical man to accomplish Full Deliverance for the spirit, the soul, and the BODY.

"20 For our conversation is in heaven; from whence also we look for the Saviour, the Lord Jesus Christ: 21 Who shall change our vile body, that it may be fashioned like unto his glorious body, according to the working whereby he is able even to subdue all things unto himself."
—Philippians 3:20-21 KJV

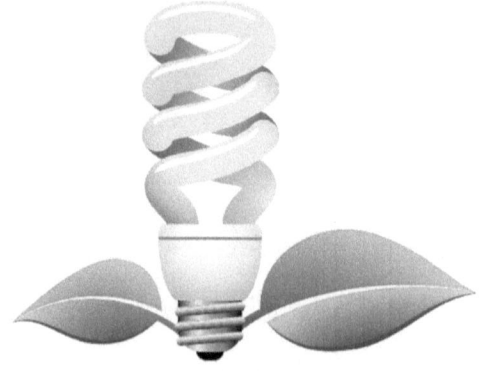

14-DAY SHIFT

This is an exciting time! You have made a conscious decision to renew and cleanse your body. During this journey, your full engagement is vital. Let's support your efforts by journaling:

- Daily Prayers
  (to include 2 Corinthians 10: 4-5)
- Thoughts and Feelings
  (*replacing every negative thought with a Godly thought*)
- Water Intake
- Food and Snack*(s)* Intake
- Retro *(7)* Minute Workouts *(daily)*

Weigh-Ins, which will be on Day 1, Day 7 and Day 14. Encouraged to take before and after pictures *(ideal, yet optional)*

NECESSARY ITEMS

- Xtreme Shaper Slimming Belt (Available on Groupon)
- Albolene Moisturizing Cleanser o (Available at Walmart, Walgreens or CVS)
- Blender *(preferably, a Nutribullet or Ninja)*
- A Notebook or Journal
- Large Cold Cup or Yeti for your smoothies

JUMP START

Hydration is important on your journey to renew and cleanse your body. A glass of **cold** Alkaline Water *(8-16 oz, not the "hyssop water")* should be consumed upon waking each day to jump start your body and metabolism. The average normal body temperature is generally 98.5 degrees, so after drinking the glass of water the body will immediately shift to burning or warming up at the start of each day. Feel free to add crystal light or sugar free flavoring, as desired.

HYSSOP WATER

Breakfast should be consumed between 6am-10:30am. This should be your cold water upon waking and the detox water (30) minutes before your smoothie (if milk is preferred, use almond, coconut, quinoa, or hemp milk. If protein powder is preferred, use plant-based powders). If you are on the go, muscle milk shakes may be an alternate for your smoothie.

Lunch should be consumed between 12noon - 3pm. This should be a sensible meal, a meat (fish or chicken, the size of your palm) and vegetables (no canned goods). If eating a salad, preferred dressings are guacamole, lemon juice, oil and vinegar or vinaigrette.

Snacks can be fruits, vegetables, or raw unsalted nuts. Try (1) cup of pecan halves and (1) Cup of dried cranberries if something sweet is desired.

Dinner should be consumed no later than 6:30pm. You can finish your left-over lunch, have a sensible meal, vegetables only or a smoothie. If having a smoothie for dinner, it must include (1) of the three: pineapples, an apple or citrus for vitamin c.

HYSSOP WATER

The "Hyssop Water" is the key component to this detox cleansing process! This water should be consumed during the entire 14 Day Shift, especially before and after each meal. Be sure to drink a glass **FIRST THING IN THE MORNING** each day at room temperature. This detox water will inspire healthier food choices, decrease sweet tooth cravings, and help with feeling full— eliminating overeating.

Drink the detox water throughout the day, consuming 1 gallon daily. Let's focus on incorporating water intake throughout the night as well, to keep the body hydrated.

Prepare a large pitcher or recycle an alkaline water jug *(24)* hours prior to starting, once the ingredients are added allow it to sit at room temperate over night for the fusing process.

See ingredients below:
1 Gallon of Alkaline or Spring Water
2 Lemons *(cut up, DO NOT squeeze)*
   Fresh Mint Leaves *(2 per sprig, use half)*
1 Tsp. to 1 ½ Tbsp. of Cayenne Pepper
   (measure to taste)
1 Cucumber

There are specific times to drink this water — *(30)* minutes before each meal and *(2)* hours after each meal. Do not add any maple syrup or agave to the pitcher/jug; you may add it to the individual glasses throughout the day, if needed. You may use Madhava Naturally Sweet Agave. However, this **may** slow down the detoxification.

MEALS

Breakfast should be consumed between 6AM-10:30AM. Before breakfast, you should drink 8oz of cold water or hyssop water (the detox water) *(30)* minutes before your breakfast or a smoothie *(if milk is preferred, use Almond, Coconut, Quinoa or Hemp Milk. If protein powder is preferred, use plant-based powders to prepare the smoothie)*, as a meal replacement. **(see smoothie recipes in the next chapter).**

If you are on the go, a Muscle Milk Shakes may be an alternate for your smoothie.

Lunch should be consumed between 12NOON-3PM. This should be a sensible meal, of a meat *(fish or chicken, the size of your palm)* and vegetables *(no canned vegetables allowed)*. If eating a salad, the preferred dressings is guacamole, lemon juice, olive oil, and vinegar or vinaigrette.

Snacks can be fruits, vegetables, or raw unsalted nuts. Try *(1)* cup of pecan halves and *(1)* cup of dried cranberries, if something sweet is desired.

Dinner should be consumed no later than 6:30PM. You can finish your left-over lunch, have a sensible meal, vegetables only or a smoothie. If having a smoothie for dinner, it must include *(1)* of the three fruits: 2oz pineapples, a regular sized apple or a regular sized citrus of choice for Vitamin C.

SMOOTHIES

Pick a Berry Smoothie

- 2 Handfuls of Kale and Arugula
- 1 Handful of your favorite berry
- 1 Handful of Blueberries
- 2 Tbsp. of Peanut Butter
- 2 Tbsp. of AquaFaba and Bladderwrack

Directions: Start with 8oz of coconut water, spring water (don't need to use alkaline water because you'll be adding the Aqua Faba) or if your preference is for a creamier consistency, use milk (recommended) Almond, Hemp, Quinoa, or Coconut. Adding the water or milk first for those who are new to smoothies the water or milk make for a better result. You can add more water or milk to perfect your smoothie to the consistency you desire.

Pineapple-Spinach Smoothie

- 2 Handfuls of Spinach
- 1 Cup of Pineapple Chunks
- 2 Cups of Peaches
- 1 Whole Banana (if large, use ½, if small use 2)
- 1 Tbsp. of Chia or Flax Seeds
- 2 Tbsp. of AquaFaba and Bladderwrack

Directions: Start with 8oz of coconut water, spring water (don't need to use alkaline water because you'll be adding the Aqua Faba) or if your preference is for a creamier consistency, use milk (recommended) Almond, Hemp, Quinoa, or Coconut. Adding the water or milk first for those who are new to smoothies the water or milk make for a better result. You can add more water or milk to perfect your smoothie to the consistency you desire.

Apple-Mango Smoothie

- 2 Handfuls of Spring Mix
- 1 ½ Mango Chunks
- 2 Cups of Strawberries
- 1 Apple
- 2 Cups of Water
- 1 Tbsp. of Chia or Flax Seeds
- 2 Tbsp. of AquaFaba and Bladderwrack

Directions: Start with 8oz of coconut water, spring water (don't need to use alkaline water because you'll be adding the Aqua Faba) or if your preference is for a creamier consistency, use milk (recommended) Almond, Hemp, Quinoa, or Coconut. Adding the water or milk first for those who are new to smoothies the water or milk make for a better result. You can add more water or milk to perfect your smoothie to the consistency you desire.

Kale Smoothie

- 2 Handfuls of Baby Kale
- 1 Beet (fresh, not canned or use organic beet power)
- 1 Cup of Pineapple Chunks
- 1 Apple
- 1 Whole Banana (if large, use ½, if small use 2)
- ½ Cup of Almond, Coconut, Quinoa or Hemp Milk
- ½ Cup of Water
- 1 Tbsp. of Chia or Flax Seeds
- 2 Tbsp. of AquaFaba and Bladderwrack

Directions: Start with 8oz of coconut water, spring water (don't need to use alkaline water because you'll be adding the Aqua Faba) or if your preference is for a creamier consistency, use milk (recommended) Almond, Hemp, Quinoa, or Coconut. Adding the water or milk first for those who are new to smoothies the water or milk make for a better result. You can add more water or milk to perfect your smoothie to the consistency you desire.

Berry-Peach Smoothie

- 2 Handfuls of Spinach
- 1 Cup of Mango Chunks
- 1 Cup of Blackberries
- 1 Apple
- 1 Handful of Seeded Grapes
- 1 Cup of Water
- 1 Cup of Almond, Coconut, Quinoa or Hemp Milk
- 2 Tbsp. of Chia or Flax Seeds
- 2 Tbsp. of AquaFaba and Bladderwrack

Directions: Start with 8oz of coconut water, spring water (don't need to use alkaline water because you'll be adding the Aqua Faba) or if your preference is for a creamier consistency, use milk (recommended) Almond, Hemp, Quinoa, or Coconut. Adding the water or milk first for those who are new to smoothies the water or milk make for a better result. You can add more water or milk to perfect your smoothie to the consistency you desire.

Berry-Berry Smoothie

- 2 Handfuls of Spring Mix
- 1 Scoop pf Beet Power
- 1 Handful of Raspberries
- 1 Handful of Strawberries
- 1 Blackberries
- 1 Apple
- 1 Whole Banana (if large use ½, if sm use 2)
- ½ Cup of Almond, Coconut, Quinoa or Hemp Milk
- ½ Cup of Water
- 1 Tbsp. of Chia or Flax Seeds
- 2 Tbsp. of AquaFaba and Bladderwrack

Directions: Start with 8oz of coconut water, spring water (don't need to use alkaline water because you'll be adding the Aqua Faba) or if your preference is for a creamier consistency, use milk (recommended) Almond, Hemp, Quinoa, or Coconut. Adding the water or milk first for those who are new to smoothies the water or milk make for a better result. You can add more water or milk to perfect your smoothie to the consistency you desire.

You Name It Smoothie

Create a smoothie and name it, then document your ingredients and measurements just like the smoothies above.

Feel free to interchange the smoothies listed above throughout the 14 Day Shift and select your favorite smoothies. Be sure to identify which smoothie gives you the most energy, keeps you full longer, etc.

Why Aquafaba?

AquaFaba is the gel form of Sea Moss that is known for boosting the immune system and metabolism. Sea Moss has 92 of the 102 vitamins and minerals that the body needs daily for those who do not eat enough leafy greens. Bladderwrack is a sea berry known for helping to improve blood circulation, vision, thyroid and suppress appetite while boosting the metabolism. This combination will improve your results for successful detoxification.

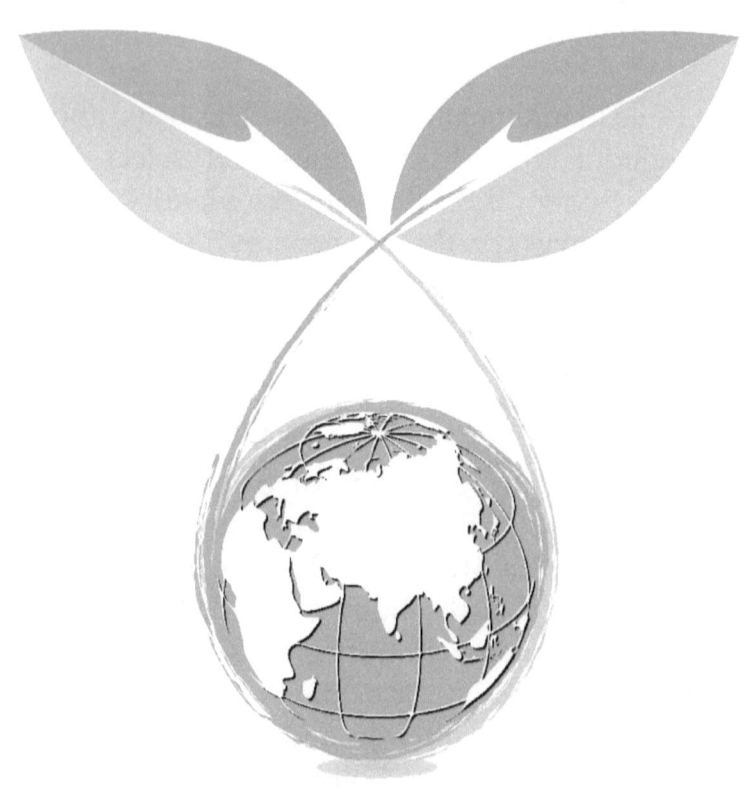

RETRO 7-MINUTE WORKOUTS

Retro 7 Minute Workouts

Think of something you did for recreation when you were younger? Something back in the day that you did not realize was a full body workout. Like dancing, roller skating, walking and bike riding. The Retro 7 Minute Workouts are just that—restoring what was once fun to do or becoming more active without the mandatory exercise perspective. This should be done for (7) minutes daily while detoxing. This activity will eventually increase in minutes as you progress, building endurance to help maintain your weight loss and tone your body.

Other examples are jump rope, bike riding, kick boxing, gardening, cutting gas, tennis, playing with children/grandchildren or household chores that require bending and squatting.

Alternative: Download the App 7 Minute Workout- HIIT for exercise routines.

Slimming Agents

These three slimming agents are a triple threat! Try either the ointment or balm to discover your preference. The Albolene Moisturizing Cleanser or the Aboniki Balm helps to mobilize fat cells rapidly to eliminate stubborn belly fat when applied topically. Make sure skin is dry. Take a quarter of a teaspoon of Albolene or a dime size of Aboniki Balm (will give an Icy Hot or Bengay effect) and rub it on your midsection and sides. Then apply the waist trainer.

The Xtreme Shaper Slimming Belt (waist trainer) should be worn each morning. As you are preparing for your day, remember your trainer. This will burn the fat from your midsection and sides even while you are in a sitting position, each movement you make will generate the heat needed in specific areas to ultimately burn fat. This should be worn for (8) hours per day.

ACCEPTABLE FOODS

Oils Grapeseed Avocado Oils
Olive Oil (only for sauces or dressings)

Seasonings

Mrs. Dash
McCormick Perfect Pinch Signature Blend
Sea Salt (limit intake) Basil

Cayenne Pepper	Cilantro
Dill	Garlic
Ginger	Oregano
Pepper	Rosemary
Sage	Thyme
Parsley	Tarragon

Meats

Trout Flounder

Mackerel	White Fish
Salmon	Cod
Sea Bass	Mahi Mahi
Halibut	Tuna

Ocean Perch Sardines
Chicken (boneless/skinless)

Vegetables

Tomatoes (Roma and Cherry)
Greens (turnips, collards, kale, chard)

Brussel Sprouts	Celery
Radishes	Asparagus
Bean Sprouts	Spinach
Cabbage	Carrots
Mushrooms	Cauliflower
Green Beans	Broccoli
Zucchini	

Lettuce (romaine, arugula, and mixed greens)

Bell Peppers	Eggplant
Onions	Okra
Squash	Peas
Cauliflower	Beets
Avocado	Bamboo Shoots
Artichoke	Olives
Bok Choy	Cucumber

Foods to Avoid: All dairy, red meats, pork (and bacon), sodas, sugars, grains including bread, cakes, pastries, pasta (anything made with flour), potatoes, corn, starchy vegetables, legumes, and anything canned or processed.

SHIFT NOW

Remember, we are aligning the triune man! The body is equally as powerful as the spirit and the soul, they each work as one with different functionalities. So, let's get ready to divinely shift to feel and look amazing.

Here is a declaration and scripture to encourage you...

"I can do all things through Christ which strengtheneth me."

Philippians 4:13 KJV

Testimonials

We welcome your feedback! Please email us and share your experience throughout this journey of physical deliverance for the body.

BIO

I am Naturopathic Practitioner who as a child of a Reverend watched my Mother medicate herself until death.

I've always known it had to be a better way to take care of the body.

It wasn't until I turned to the Bible where I was inspired to look deeper as to why God says Spirit, Mind, and Body. I took the simplicity of what the Bible has given as tools to begin bringing the body to an alkaline state.

CONNECT WITH ME

Connect with me on
Facebook @ Return 2 Divinity: Fit for the Kingdom
Email @ return2divinitywc@gmail.com
To Purchase the AquaFaba and Bladderwrack,
Send Payments to PayPal @ Yg40@hotmail.com
CashApp @ $DrYoR2D
Cost: $75.00